THE ENCYCLOPEDIA OF VISUAL MEDICINE SERIES

A Slide Atlas of ECHOCARDIOGRAPHY

John Chambers MD, FRCP, FACC
Senior Lecturer and Consultant in Cardiology
Guy's Hospital and St. Thomas' Hospital
London, UK

The Parthenon Publishing Group
International Publishers in Medicine, Science & Technology
NEW YORK LONDON

Published in the USA by:
The Parthenon Publishing Group Inc., One Blue Hill Plaza, PO Box 1564, Pearl River, New York 10965, USA
Tel: (914) 735 9363 Fax: (914) 735 1385

Published in the UK and Europe by:
The Parthenon Publishing Group Limited, Casterton Hall, Carnforth, Lancs. LA6 2LA, UK
Tel: 44 (0) 15242 72084 Fax: 44 (0) 15242 71587

ISBN: 1-85070-958-0

Captions to Slides

The normal heart

Slide 1 *Ultrasound windows* Ultrasound access to the heart is constrained by the ribs and lungs to small 'windows' of which the parasternal and apical windows are the most frequently used. The right intercostal and suprasternal windows are used for imaging the aorta and the substernal window for imaging the inferior vena cava and atrial septum

Slide 2 *Normal parasternal long-axis view* Most studies start with the parasternal long-axis view. The papillary muscles (1) are attached via the chordae (2) to the anterior (3) and posterior (4) mitral leaflets. The mitral annulus consists of a fibrous mitral-aortic intervalve fibrosa (5) anteriorly and a non-fibrous portion (6) at the junction with the left atrium laterally and posteriorly. The left, non-coronary (7) and right coronary (8) cusps of the aortic valve can be seen opening towards the sinus of Valsalva (9)

Slide 3 *Normal short-axis view at aortic valve level* Further views are taken with the transducer turned 90° clockwise. The heart can then be scanned from virtually the apex up to the base of the heart. Three conventional views are recorded. The first is at aortic valve level and is used for imaging movement of the aortic valve. The right heart can be seen 'embracing' the aorta, with right atrium, right ventricle and pulmonary artery in clockwise order

Slide 4 *Normal short-axis view at mitral valve level* The next standard section is at mitral valve level. The right ventricle can easily be seen as a crescentic structure anterior and to the right of the left ventricle. The left ventricle should be circular and flattening of the septum suggests right ventricular dilatation or pulmonary hypertension. The mitral valve orifice should span virtually the entire width of the left ventricular cavity

Slide 5 *Normal short-axis view of the left ventricle* The final conventional parasternal short-axis view is at papillary muscle level. This shows regions supplied by all three main epicardial coronary arteries and is particularly useful for localizing wall motion abnormalities

Slide 6 *Normal four-chamber view* Imaging in the apical window starts with the 'four-chamber' view. Angling inferiorly shows the inferior septum supplied by the posterior descending artery and the postero-lateral wall supplied by the circumflex artery. Angling upwards shows the aorta in the 'five-chamber' view which is used for recording pulsed Doppler in the left ventricular outflow tract. The 'four-chamber' view is used for recording transmitral pulsed Doppler with the sample volume level with the tips of the mitral leaflets in their fully open diastolic position. Rotation of the transducer allows 'two-chamber' and apical long-axis views

Slide 7 *M-mode of left ventricle and aorta/left atrium* Measurements of cavity size on M-mode imaging are made with the cursor positioned just below the tips of the mitral leaflets in the parasternal short- or long-axis view. Diastolic dimensions are taken by convention on the Q wave. The smallest diameter is taken for the left ventricular systolic dimension. The aorta is also measured on the Q wave while the largest left atrial diameter possible is taken. All measurements are taken by convention from leading edge to leading edge. s, septal width; pw, posterior wall width; sd, systolic LV diameter; dd, diastolic LV diameter; Ao, aortic diameter; LA, left aortal diameter

Slide 8 *M-mode of the mitral valve* M-mode recordings of the mitral valve may sometimes help in the diagnosis of rheumatic mitral disease or mitral prolapse. The mitral leaflets open (1) at the start of early fast filling (E). The leaflets then drift towards the closed position (2) during diastasis (D) before opening again during atrial systole (A). After this, the leaflets drift closed (3)

Valve disease – aortic

Slide 9 *Calcific degenerative disease* This image shows a heavily thickened valve from the parasternal long-axis (a) and short-axis view (b) during systole. The valve cusps have hardly moved from their closed position in diastole. Echocardiography cannot reliably differentiate the various etiologies of aortic valve disease (calcific degeneration, bicuspid valve or rheumatic disease) when the valve has become significantly calcified

Slide 10 *M-mode in moderate aortic stenosis* Thickening of the cusps and reduced excursion in systole are readily seen

Slide 11 *Bicuspid aortic valve* The larger of the two cusps has a median raphe (arrow) representing the unseparated cusp edges

Slide 12 *M-mode of normal (a) and bicuspid aortic valve (b)* The pathognomonic feature is the eccentric closure line (arrowed). In addition, the bicuspid valve is thickened and has reduced excursion in systole. On two-dimensional imaging, the valve domes during systole

Slide 13 *Rheumatic aortic valve* This abnormality is characterized by thickening of the valve with doming during systole but with a central closure line. On the short-axis view, three cusps of equal size can be seen. In addition, it is common to have coexistent thickening of the mitral valve. Rheumatic disease tends to be associated with greater regurgitation than calcific degenerative disease as a result of retraction of the cusp tips

Slide 14 *Aortic dilatation* Aortic regurgitation is caused by abnormalities of the ascending aorta or of the valve or both. Aortic dilatation, as shown here, is usually caused by medial necrosis as a result of age or hypertension. Occasionally, it is associated with collagen diseases such as Marfan syndrome or with aortic dissection

Slide 15 *Aortic valve prolapse* Movement of a part of one or more cusps behind the line of the echocardiographic annulus is called prolapse. This may accompany mitral valve prolapse. Other causes of aortic regurgitation are diaphenous aortic valve (a condition in which the valve becomes thin without calcifying) and endocarditis

Slide 16 *Quantification of aortic stenosis* The modified Bernoulli theorem states that the sum of potential and kinetic energy on either side of a stenotic valve must remain equal. If the pressure P falls across a stenotic valve, the kinetic energy must rise. ρ is the density of blood and $\frac{1}{2}\rho$ for blood at body temperature is approximately 4. The subaortic velocity can be omitted provided that it is much less than the transaortic velocity. This is not the case for mild aortic stenosis (peak velocity less than 3 m/s) or for normally functioning aortic prostheses. The equation can be used to assess the severity of a stenotic valve lesion and to estimate pulmonary artery pressure and the pressure difference across a ventricular septal defect

Slide 17 *Continuous wave recording in aortic stenosis* This signal was recorded from the apex in a patient with severe aortic stenosis. The signal has been planimetered, giving a semi-automated read-out of peak and also mean pressure difference. In this example, the peak subaortic velocity of 1 m/s was trivial and thus excluded from the modified Bernoulli theorem. The peak velocity of 4.7 m/s then gives an estimated maximum gradient of 90 mmHg. The mean gradient is always more representative than the peak since it is calculated using the whole waveform. In this case, the mean gradient is displayed as 53.8 mmHg which should be rounded up to 55 mmHg

Slide 18 *Comparison of Doppler ultrasound and catheter-estimated pressure drop* Doppler ultrasound measures the true peak instantaneous difference in pressure across the aortic valve. At catheterization, it is usual to pull the catheter back across the aortic valve, giving a 'pull-back' or 'peak-to-peak' gradient which is usually less than the Doppler gradient by around 20 mmHg. However, this difference may vary between 0 and 50 mmHg. The catheter gradient is not a true physiological pressure difference, as the peaks on the aortic and left ventricular pressure waveforms do not occur simultaneously. Furthermore, the pressure downstream from the valve tends to rise progressively beyond the valve, so the catheter effectively measures the pressure difference between the left ventricle and the aorta rather than across the aortic valve

Slide 19 *Theory of the continuity equation* Pressure gradients are highly dependent on flow. A gradient of 30 mmHg can be obtained in mild aortic stenosis at high flow or in a patient with severe aortic stenosis at low cardiac output. For this reason, flow correction is usually necessary if the gradient is low or moderate in the presence of a poor left ventricle. The most widespread method of flow correction is the continuity equation. This is based on the law of conservation of mass which states that the volume of flow below the aortic valve must be the same as the volume of flow through the aortic valve. Therefore, the product of cross-sectional area below the valve and the subaortic velocity integral (the planimetered area of the subaortic pulsed Doppler signal) must be the same as the effective orifice area of the aortic valve times the velocity integral of the continuous wave transaortic signal. Assuming that the subaortic and transaortic waveforms are of the same shape, it is usual to simplify the calculation by using peak velocity instead of the velocity integral. Thus the continuity equation becomes: effective orifice area (EOA) of A_2 = cross-sectional area of left ventricular outflow tract (A_1) times subaortic peak velocity (v_1) divided by transaortic peak velocity (v_2)

Slide 20 *Application of the continuity equation* In this example, the aortic valve was heavily calcified, but, because the left ventricle was severely impaired, the transaortic peak velocity was only 2.5 m/s. The subaortic diameter was 2.1 cm, giving a cross-sectional outflow tract area of 3.5 cm^2. The subaortic peak velocity was 0.5 m/s, giving an effective orifice area of 3.5 times 0.5 divided by 2.5, or 0.7 cm^2. This suggests severe stenosis

Slide 21 *The left ventricle and aortic stenosis* A high pressure gradient leads to left ventricular hypertrophy as a compensatory mechanism to reduce wall stress. Initially, cardiac output is maintained, but at the cost of increasing diastolic dysfunction. Ultimately, subendocardial fibrosis may supervene, leading to systolic dysfunction. The mortality when heart failure develops is 50% at 1 year

Slide 22 *Signs of severity in aortic stenosis*

Slide 23 *Color flow mapping in aortic regurgitation* The degree of aortic regurgitation is determined by the driving pressure across the aortic valve in diastole, by the size of the regurgitant orifice and by other factors such as the compliance of the left ventricle and heart rate. The size of the regurgitant orifice correlates reasonably well with the height of the jet expressed as a percentage of the height of the left ventricular outflow tract. This is a patient with severe aortic regurgitation in whom the jet fills the left ventricular outflow tract

Slide 24 *Mild aortic regurgitation* This is a thin jet in a patient with mild aortic regurgitation. The jet height is less than 25% of the height of the outflow tract

Slide 25 *Continuous wave Doppler in aortic regurgitation* In severe aortic regurgitation, the aortic and left ventricular pressures approximate towards the end of diastole. The pressure difference across the valve is, therefore, small and the end-diastolic velocity correspondingly low. This leads to a steep descent of the diastolic signal (a). At the same time, the forward flow velocity is usually high and the signal tends to be dense. In more moderate aortic regurgitation (b), the signal has a gentler slope and the peak forward flow velocity is lower

Slide 26 *Color flow reversal in diastole in the aorta* The more severe the regurgitation, the further down the aorta can flow reversal be detected and the longer it lasts during diastole. In this example, in a patient with severe regurgitation, color reversal can be seen as far as the descending thoracic aorta (right). On color M-mode (left), reversal shown in red lasts throughout diastole

Slide 27 *The left ventricle in aortic regurgitation* The left ventricle is dilated and hyperkinetic as a result of the large filling volumes. Dilated left ventricles have a high wall stress and eccentric hypertrophy develops as a compensatory mechanism. A fall in fractional shortening may be a sign of left ventricular decompensation and, as an approximate rule of thumb, recovery after aortic valve surgery may not occur if the fractional shortening falls below 25%

Slide 28 *Signs of severity in aortic regurgitation*

Valve disease – mitral

Slide 29 *Rheumatic disease of the mitral valve* There is elbowing of the base of the anterior leaflet during diastole with thickening at the tips of the leaflets. There may be involvement of the chordae. Balloon valvotomy is contraindicated in the presence of dense matting of the chordae, as in this example, or thickening and immobility of the base of the anterior leaflet, or in the presence of more than mild mitral regurgitation or a left atrial thrombus

Slide 30 *M-mode of a rheumatic mitral valve* The features are the thickened leaflet tips (1) with reduced excursion of the anterior leaflet (2), anterior rather than posterior diastolic motion of the posterior leaflet (3) as a result of commissural fusion, and finally, slow filling of the left ventricle (4). In this example, there is also vibration of the septum (5) from an impinging jet of aortic regurgitation

Slide 31 *Mitral prolapse* This is an apical 'four-chamber' view. Curvature of the posterior leaflet above the plane of the annulus during systole can be seen in the left-hand panel with a broad jet of mitral regurgitation directed anteriorly (right-hand panel)

Slide 32 *Mitral valve endocarditis* A large echogenic mass is attached to the mitral valve but moves out of phase with the leaflets, prolapsing into the left atrium in systole (a) and into the left ventricle in diastole (b). This is a classical vegetation

Slide 33 *Functional mitral regurgitation* Left ventricular dilatation causing a change in the angle of the papillary muscles relative to the mitral valve can cause anything from mild to severe mitral regurgitation. In this case, the left ventricular dilatation was caused by chronic severe aortic regurgitation

Slide 34 *Restricted mitral valve in ischemic disease* There is a posterior myocardial infarction. This means that the normal piston-like movement of the annulus towards the apex during systole is reduced. The posterior leaflet is therefore unable to rest back towards the annulus during systole causing failure of apposition (arrow). The jet of mitral regurgitation is directed posteriorly. This type of mitral regurgitation may be corrected by mitral annuloplasty

Slide 35 *Continuous wave Doppler in mitral stenosis* Velocities are raised throughout diastole but are highly dependent on the length of the cycle. The end-diastolic velocity is almost normal on the second complex (A) but it is 1.6 m/s on the third (B). The slope of the signal, however, is approximately constant, despite changing cycle lengths. The pressure half-time is the time taken for the peak pressure difference to halve. Because pressure drop is related to the square of velocity, this becomes the time for the peak velocity (V_{max}) to fall to $1/\sqrt{2}$ of its original value ($1/\sqrt{2} = 0.7$)

Slide 36 *Pressure half-time* The pressure half-time is a measure of the rate of descent of the velocity during diastole. It can be used to determine mitral orifice area by an empirical formula: mitral orifice area = 220/pressure half-time. This formula should only be applied in moderate or severe mitral stenosis. In mild mitral stenosis, or with a normal mitral valve, the rate of descent reflects left ventricular factors and loading conditions better than it does the state of the mitral valve

Slide 37 *Estimation of pulmonary artery systolic pressure* The pressure difference between the right ventricle and right atrium is estimated using the short form of the modified Bernoulli equation applied to the peak velocity of the tricuspid regurgitant jet. To this must be added an estimate of right atrial pressure from the percentage collapse of the inferior vena cava on inspiration. It is assumed that there is no pulmonary stenosis. In this patient, there is severe mitral stenosis with a pressure half-time >350 ms (left). Surprisingly, the patient is still in sinus rhythm. The right-hand panel shows the tricuspid signal (note the low forward flow velocities). The peak velocity of the tricuspid regurgitant signal is 4.0 m/s giving a transtricuspid pressure difference of about 65 mmHg. The inferior vena cava collapsed by 25–50%, suggesting a right atrial pressure of 15 mmHg and therefore a pulmonary artery systolic pressure of 80 mmHg

Slide 38 *Estimation of right atrial pressure*

Slide 39 *Criteria of severity in mitral stenosis*

Slide 40 *Severe mitral regurgitation* Regurgitant flow consists of a flow recruitment area in the left ventricle, then a neck passing through the mitral valve, and finally an intra-atrial jet. Clear flow recruitment, a broad neck around 1 cm in width and an intra-atrial jet greater than 8 cm^2 in area suggest severe mitral regurgitation

Slide 41 *Mild mitral regurgitation* There is no flow recruitment area. The neck is narrow and the intra-atrial jet area is less than 4 cm^2 in area. Other ways of assessing severity are from the density of the continuous wave signal and from the behavior of pulmonary vein flow. Blunting of systolic forward flow occurs with moderate mitral regurgitation and flow reversal during systole in the presence of severe mitral regurgitation

Slide 42 *The left ventricle and mitral regurgitation* In chronic severe mitral regurgitation, irreversible fibrosis of the myocardium can supervene such that subsequent mitral valve surgery does not affect long-term outcome. This deterioration is disguised because systolic function on the echocardiogram remains good until a late stage. This is because the left ventricle contracts partly into the left atrium, which is a low-pressure chamber, so afterload is low. As a rule of thumb, a fractional shortening less than 29% or an end-systolic volume of 90 ml/m^2 suggests that irreversible fibrosis has occurred. In this example, the fractional shortening before mitral surgery (a) was 29%, but this had fallen to only 15% after surgery (b)

Slide 43 *Signs of severity in mitral regurgitation*

Valve disease – prosthetic valves

Slide 44 *Prosthetic valves* The valves are all shown in 'four-chamber' views. (a) Porcine bioprosthesis with a strut (s), inside which a cuspal echo (arrow) can be seen; (b) a caged ball prosthesis with a sewing ring (sr), cage (c) and ball (arrow); (c) tilting disk valve with sewing ring (sr) and disk (arrow); (d) bileaflet prosthesis with sewing ring (sr) and two leaflets (arrowed)

Slide 45 *Sign of failing biological valve* The cusps of most biological valves on echocardiography are 1 mm thick. They are considered abnormal if greater than 3 mm in thickness. In this example of a bovine pericardial valve, the upper leaflet is normal, whereas the lower leaflet is thickened. Thickening of the echo may reflect minor tears in the cusp margin and is associated with severe primary failure in around 40% of cases within 2 years

Slide 46 *Abnormal occluder motion* In mechanical valves in the mitral position, reduced or abnormal motion of the leaflets or ball are signs of obstruction. In this case, in a patient with a bileaflet prosthesis, the laterally placed leaflet is fully open (arrow) whilst the more medial leaflet is fixed in the closed position

Slide 47 *Obstruction in the mitral prosthesis on continuous wave Doppler* The pressure half-time does not reliably reflect orifice area since it is partly determined by left ventricular diastolic behavior and loading conditions. However, in a significantly obstructed valve, the pressure half-time is markedly prolonged. In this example, the pressure half-time rose from 55 ms (A) to 350 ms (B) when the valve became obstructed by thrombus. Pressure half-times longer than 200 ms are likely to be abnormal

Slide 48 *Criteria of obstruction in a mitral prosthesis* Other helpful signs suggesting obstruction are a narrow color flow profile, a rise in pulmonary artery pressures and slow left ventricular filling. The single most useful sign is usually abnormal motion of the cusps or occluder. A prolonged pressure half-time, if associated with high peak velocities greater than 2.5 m/s, then makes the diagnosis almost certain

Slide 49 *Suspicion of obstruction in an aortic prosthesis* Obstruction is relatively less likely in a mechanical aortic prosthesis since thrombosis is less likely to occur than in the mitral position. Furthermore, high transaortic velocities can be recorded in normally functioning valves, particularly if these are small, of annulus diameter 19 mm or 21 mm. In an asymptomatic patient, obstruction should not be overdiagnosed. High velocities should always be compared against normal ranges for the specific annulus diameter and valve design. The variation is too great to allow unitary thresholds for abnormality. However, an effective orifice area by the continuity equation of less than 1 cm^2 is suspicious of obstruction in valves greater than size 21 mm. It is important to perform a post-operative study when the valve can be assumed to be working normally, and a fall in the effective orifice area by more than 30% is then suspicious of obstruction. The velocity ratio is the ratio of the subaortic peak velocity to the transaortic peak velocity. This can be used for serial studies in the same valve since the left ventricular outflow tract cross-sectional area can be assumed to be constant. A velocity ratio less than 0.2 suggests obstruction

Slide 50 *Regurgitation in mechanical valves* Most mechanical valves are designed to have a closing volume (A) which pulls the occluder shut and after this true leakage occurs around the occluder (B). Bileaflet valves have leakage at the pivotal points. The regurgitant fraction can be around 10% and the jets can look surprisingly large on color flow mapping. They have to be distinguished from abnormal paraprosthetic leaks

Slide 51 *Normal pivotal washing jets in a bileaflet prosthesis in the aortic position* In the aortic position, it is possible to see normal transprosthetic regurgitation in most mechanical valves. These are usually of low momentum and usually relatively narrow at their base. There are characteristic patterns for each design of valve, for example, single tilting disc valves have two jets, one from the minor and one from major orifice. Bileaflet valves have jets either side of each pivotal point, as shown in this example. There are two red jets from the lower and two in blue/green from the upper pivotal point

Slide 52 *Paraprosthetic aortic regurgitation* By contrast, a paraprosthetic jet has its origin outside the sewing ring and there is no relationship with the known structure of the valve. The degree of paraprosthetic regurgitation can be assessed using conventional methods as applied to the native valve. However, the width of the jet in relation to the left ventricular outflow tract height is less reliable since the jet may be eccentric. Another method available is to assess the proportion of the circumference of the sewing ring occupied by the jet. This example shows a large jet occupying about 30% of the circumference

Slide 53 *Transprosthetic and paraprosthetic regurgitation in the mitral position* It is rare to see normal transprosthetic regurgitation in mitral valves using transthoracic echocardiography. If jets are seen, these are almost always paraprosthetic even though their origin may be difficult to define because of shielding by the mechanical parts of the valve. Transesophageal echocardiography is necessary if such jets are shown or if the patient is symptomatic or has a murmur, even despite a normal transthoracic study. In this example, two low momentum pivotal washing jets can be seen in the center of the valve with a much larger paraprosthetic jet with its origin clearly outside the sewing ring

Endocarditis

Slide 54 *Vegetations* The vegetation is the hallmark of endocarditis. Classically, it is a mobile echogenic mass attached to the valve and moving out of phase with that valve. In this example, there are vegetations (arrows) attached to both aortic and mitral valves in a patient with hypertrophic cardiomyopathy

Slide 55 *Number of vegetations detected* Transthoracic echocardiography has approximately a 60% sensitivity for the detection of vegetations compared with approximately 90% sensitivity on transesophageal echocardiography. However, the sensitivity depends on the size of the vegetation and on the valve disease present. Most vegetations greater than 10 mm in diameter can be found even on transthoracic echocardiography. Transesophageal echocardiography is necessary to detect vegetations on mechanical replacement valves in most cases

Slide 56 *Perforation* Endocarditis is also shown by the presence of valve destruction causing valve regurgitation and by complications including perforation which in this example is seen in the anterior mitral leaflet

Slide 57 *Abscess* Other local complications of endocarditis are dehiscence of a prosthetic valve, fistula and abscess. The left-hand panel shows thickening of the aortic root on a transthoracic study. The transesophageal study in the same patient shows a characteristic septated cavity (arrow) in the posterior part of the aortic root

Slide 58 *Complications in endocarditis* Complications are more likely to be found on transesophageal echocardiography, particularly when endocarditis occurs on a prosthetic valve. However, the two techniques are complementary since anterior aortic root abscesses may show only transthoracically

Slide 59 *The equivocal mass* Echocardiography can only be interpreted adequately in the clinical context. Classical vegetations may not always be found and the likelihood of a mass being a vegetation depends on the clinical likelihood of endocarditis. Furthermore, vegetations may remain even after successful treatment and do not indicate active infection. In this case, echoes attached to the anterior mitral leaflet were found incidentally in an asymptomatic patient. Full investigation showed no evidence of endocarditis and the echoes were interpreted as redundant chordae

Ischemic disease including left ventricular function

Slide 60 *The arterial supply of the heart* This is shown in parasternal short-axis (a), long-axis (b) and 'four-chamber' (c) views. Transverse short-axis views are the single best views for monitoring left ventricular function since they show the territories of all three major epicardial arteries. l, left anterior descending; c, circumflex; r, right coronary

Slide 61 *Regional motion scores* Regional motion scores can be given to every segment of the left ventricle in which at least 50% of the endocardium is visible. For clinical use, inward motion of the endocardium should be described qualitatively for each arterial territory

Slide 62 *Regional hypokinesis* There is inferior infarction shown as a bulging region (arrowed in left panel). The M-mode recording at this level confirms that the posterior wall thickens little during systole. There is compensatory hyperkinesis of the septum which means that global function assessed by ejection fraction or stroke volume can be near normal even with obvious regional wall motion abnormalities. Lack of compensatory hyperkinesis is a sign of multivessel coronary disease

Slide 63 *Regional dyskinesis* In this patient with an anterior myocardial infarction, the apex and adjacent septum are thin and move paradoxically, i.e. outwards in systole (right, arrows) when the rest of the left ventricle is moving inwards. D, diastole; S, systole

Slide 64 *Global function* Some measure of global function should also be assessed, either end-systolic volume, ejection fraction or stroke volume. In this example, the end-systolic endocardial border has been traced and the volume calculated assuming regular geometry. The normal end-systolic volume ranges up to 67 ml in a male and 57 ml in a female. End-systolic frames are usually easy to measure. Ejection fraction can be calculated from the difference between end-diastolic and end-systolic volumes, divided by the end-diastolic volume and expressed as a percentage. This is relatively inaccurate and only an approximate range can be given

Slide 65 *Estimation of stroke volume* This can be calculated from the product of the cross-sectional area of the left ventricular outflow tract (calculated from the diameter, d, assuming circular geometry) and the area of the subaortic signal, recorded using pulsed Doppler methods – this is the stroke distance or systolic velocity integral. A 15% change in stroke volume can be detected with 95% certainty using Doppler ultrasound

Slide 66 *Diastolic left ventricular function* Transmitral pulsed Doppler recordings can be used to describe left ventricular diastolic behavior. Early velocity (E) is succeeded by a period of diastasis and finally by atrial systole (A). The deceleration time of the E wave is measured from the peak of the wave to the point at which it meets the baseline (a). This is normally 140–280 ms. A similar measurement can be made for the A wave. This is normally greater than 70 ms. Two basic abnormal patterns exist. The slow relaxation pattern (b) is characterized by a low E velocity with a prolonged E wave deceleration time and an augmented A velocity. This is typically found in patients with left ventricular hypertrophy. A restrictive pattern (c) is characterized by a tall E wave, short E deceleration time and small or absent A wave. This is found in restrictive myopathy or in any condition associated with high filling pressures and/or a rapid rise in left ventricular diastolic pressure, for example, pericardial constriction

Slide 67 *Criteria for abnormal left ventricular function*

Slide 68 *Left ventricular aneurysm* Aneurysms develop in approximately 10% of all myocardial infarctions and are associated with a survival at 1 year of around 50%

Slide 69 *Left ventricular pseudoaneurysm* A pseudoaneurysm (PAn) usually complicates an inferior infarction. It is distinguished from a true aneurysm by the presence of a narrow rather than a wide neck. Blood flows into the pseudoaneurysm during systole and out in diastole

Slide 70 *Ventricular septal rupture* There is an anterior myocardial infarction with flow from left to right ventricle across the septum. This complication occurs in 1–2% of acute infarctions

Slide 71 *Papillary muscle rupture* The postero-medial papillary muscle has partially ruptured (2). The antero-lateral muscle is intact (1). This complication occurs in 1–2% of all acute infarcts and in 5% of all fatal infarctions

Slide 72 *Papillary muscle dysfunction* Lesser degrees of mitral regurgitation occur after myocardial infarction, either as a result of ventricular dilatation, failure of the inferior wall to contract during systole leading to restriction of the posterior leaflet motion (see Slide 34), or, finally, as a result of reduced support for the posterior leaflet leading to prolapse (arrowed)

Slide 73 *Thrombus* This develops in approximately 30–40% of anterior infarctions and 3% of inferior infarcts. There is a higher rate of thromboembolism, around 15%, if a thrombus is detected, and this is probably halved by anticoagulating with warfarin

Cardiomyopathies

Slide 74 *Hypertrophic cardiomyopathy* Hypertrophy can occur anywhere within either ventricle but most frequently affects the septum. The granularity in this example is typical. Systolic function is initially preserved. Because of the reduced cavity size, the anterior mitral leaflet impinges on the septum, leading to thickening of the tip (solid arrow). Outflow acceleration causing turbulence in the outflow tract leads to thickening of the aortic valve (open arrow) which may become regurgitant. Cavity obliteration during systole is associated with premature closure of the aortic valve

Slide 75 *M mode in hypertrophic cardiomyopathy* Systolic anterior motion (arrow) is probably caused by abnormal papillary muscle function. This image also shows crowding of the mitral valve within the small left ventricular cavity. The septum is thick but contraction is preserved

Slide 76 *Dynamic flow acceleration* During systole, as the cavity shrinks, flow in the outflow tract accelerates producing a characteristic dagger shape

Slide 77 *Dilated cardiomyopathy* Global dilatation without hypertrophy is clearly shown in (left-hand panel) and on the systolic freeze-frame on two-dimensional imaging (right-hand panel). These echocardiographic appearances are non-specific and cannot differentiate most causes of a dilated left ventricle, including alcohol, myocarditis, and primary dilated myopathy

Slide 78 *Primary restrictive myopathy* Restrictive physiology is associated with left ventricular dysfunction from many causes. Restrictive myopathy is a term given to myopathies associated with a fast rate of rise of left ventricular diastolic pressure. Of these, infiltrations, notably amyloid, are the most frequent in the UK, although they still remain rare. Primary restrictive myopathy is characterized by restrictive physiology with little or no hypertrophy, no cavity dilatation, and reduced contractility. A characteristic sign is biatrial enlargement. This sign may also occur with apical hypertrophic myopathy or combined mitral and tricuspid valve disease

Slide 79 *Transmitral pulsed Doppler recording in restrictive myopathy* There is a tall E wave and virtually absent A wave with a short E wave deceleration time, below 100 ms. This is in keeping with the restrictive physiology and can occur in constrictive pericarditis as well as restrictive myopathy. However, there is virtually no respiratory variability, which is a feature of restrictive myopathy. In constrictive pericarditis, there would be an exaggerated fall in E wave velocity during inspiration. Other characteristic differentiating features are reduced left ventricular systolic function which is a feature of restrictive myopathy, whereas, in constrictive pericarditis, systolic function is normal. On superior vena cava flow, constrictive pericarditis is characterized by exaggerated flow reversal during expiration compared with exaggerated flow reversal during inspiration in restrictive myopathy. Restrictive myopathy is also associated with a prominent diastolic forward flow pattern, whereas the pattern in constrictive pericarditis may be variable

Slide 80 *Constrictive pericarditis on M-mode* Systolic function is normal. However, diastolic filling finishes early (1). There is also characteristic beaking during late systole (2) and early diastole (3), probably resulting from equalization of pressure across the two ventricles

Slide 81 *Pulsed Doppler recording in constrictive pericarditis* There is increased respiratory variability with an abnormal fall (>30%) from expiration (Ee) to inspiration (Ei) on the mitral signal (bottom panel). At the same time, aortic flow (top panel) disappears during inspiration

Pericardial effusion

Slide 82 *Pericardial versus pleural effusion* The pericardium is attached to the aorta and pulmonary veins so a pericardial effusion ends anterior (arrow) to the descending aorta while a pleural effusion ends posteriorly. Second, a pleural effusion may extend over the left atrium, but a pericardial effusion does not to any significant degree. A pericardial effusion can be approximately described by size: small (less than 1 cm), moderate (1–2 cm) and large (greater than 2 cm). However, more important is whether it is causing tamponade. This may happen even with a small but acute effusion. Conversely, a large, slowly forming effusion may cause little hemodynamic embarrassment

Slide 83 *Right ventricular collapse* Right atrial collapse is a non-specific sign showing even with small pericardial effusions. The right ventricular outflow tract is the first part of the right ventricle to show diastolic inward motion. As the hemodynamic effects of the effusion increase, collapse extends over progressively more of the right ventricular wall and lasts for progressively longer during diastole. In this illustration there is extensive collapse of the free wall between systole (b) and diastole (a). M-mode (c) shows that this lasts throughout diastole (arrow)

Slide 84 *Engorged inferior vena cava* Other signs of tamponade are an engorged inferior vena cava (greater than 2 cm in diameter) which collapses less than 25% during inspiration (normally greater than 50%), exaggeration of the inspiratory fall in transmitral E wave to greater than 40% and an abnormal superior vena cava flow pattern with forward flow predominantly in systole

Slide 85 *Normal vena cava* By comparison, a normal vena cava is less than 2 cm in diameter and contracts by > 50% between expiration (a) and inspiration (b). This is also shown in M-mode (c)

Aortic disease

Slide 86 *Aortic dissection, transthoracic view* This image shows a dissection flap beginning just above the aortic valve in parasternal (a) and transverse (b) views. The M-mode recording clearly shows a double wall caused by the upper part of the flap (large arrow) and the serpentine motion of the main part of the flap within the lumen (marked by three arrows). The sensitivity of transthoracic echocardiography is around 50% for dissections involving the ascending thoracic aorta

Slide 87 *Artefact in aorta* Reverberation artefact, usually from calcification within the aortic wall, is common and easily mistaken for a dissection flap. The flap-like structure in this example moves regularly and can be seen to mirror the right ventricular wall on the M-mode recording. Parasternal long-axis view (a) and M-mode recording (b) are shown

Slide 88 *Type B dissection on transthoracic echocardiography* A dissection is classified as type A if it involves the ascending aorta and type B if it only involves the descending aorta. Type A dissections are usually treated with immediate surgery while type B dissections are initially treated medically. The sensitivity for transthoracic echocardiography for the detection of type B dissections is around 30%

Slide 89 *Transesophageal echo in type A dissection* The hallmark of dissection is the flap dividing the true from the false lumen. The true lumen can be identified because it increases in diameter during systole and flow can easily be detected within it. In the false lumen, flow is either absent, reversed or delayed. In this example, a small subsidiary entry tear can be seen marked by blue

Slide 90 *Mural hematoma* About 10% of patients with a history suggesting acute dissection have no flap. However, the aortic wall is increased beyond its normal thickness (4 mm) and mixed echogenicity in planes can be seen. This appearance is diagnostic of a mural hematoma thought to be caused by rupture of vasa vasora. A proportion of such cases subsequently develop a dissection flap and so should be treated as for an established dissection

Slide 91 *Aortic ectasia* This is caused by medial necrosis, usually as a result of age, but with a contribution from hypertension. In a small number of cases, there is an underlying collagen abnormality, e.g. Marfan syndrome or Ehlers-Danlos type IV. In this example, medial necrosis was associated with a bicuspid aortic valve which had been replaced with a bioprosthesis 7 years before significant aortic root dilatation developed. Parasternal short- (a) and long-axis (b) views are illustrated

Slide 92 *Aortic atheroma* This is a transesophageal image in the descending aorta. Atheroma greater than 5 mm in depth, or if pedunculated (as in this example) or ulcerated have a relative risk of around 7 of causing peripheral embolization, especially after cardiac catheterization. They are found in approximately 10% of patients after cerebral infarction compared with approximately 3% in normal control subjects

Congenital disease

Slide 93 *Atrial septal defect* This parasternal short-axis view shows a dilated right ventricle which is often the first clue to the diagnosis. Flow across the atrial septum can be seen in this or, more easily, the subcostal or an off-axis apical view. It is important to differentiate it from superior vena cava flow by paying careful attention to the origin of the flow pattern. In this example, both the superior vena cava and atrial septal flow can be seen. If there is doubt, the pulsed Doppler recording in atrial septal defect shows a biphasic wave form with a late systolic peak and a diastolic peak occurring after atrial systole. In the superior vena cava, the systolic and diastolic peaks are earlier in the cardiac cycle. The shunt size can be calculated as the ratio of pulmonary to aortic stroke volume. An atrial septal defect at the fossa ovalis (secundum atrial septal defect), as in this example, is the most common congenital defect found in adults

Slide 94 *Ventricular septal defect* These are the most common congenital anomalies in children and the most common of these are perimembranous. Other defects are supracristal (straddling the aortic and pulmonary valves), inlet or muscular in location. In this image, a defect just under the aortic valve can be seen. The continuous wave recording at the left sternal edge, where the murmur is loudest, shows high velocity flow towards the transducer. The peak velocity can be used to calculate the interventricular pressure difference and, if this is subtracted from the cuff systolic pressure, it gives an estimate of pulmonary artery systolic pressure

Slide 95 *Tetralogy of Fallot* There is an overriding aorta with muscular ventricular septal defect. Right ventricular hypertrophy can be seen, although the fourth component, right ventricular outflow obstruction, is not visible

Slide 96 *Persistent ductus arteriosus* The duct is a normal developmental feature, diverting blood from the pulmonary to the systemic circulation *in utero*. It is usually closed completely by 21 days after birth. An uncomplicated persistent duct can be identified from suprasternal recordings or from the parasternal short-axis position where flow into the left pulmonary branch or, less commonly, the main pulmonary artery, can be imaged in both diastole (A) and systole (B). On continuous wave recording, there is high velocity flow throughout the cardiac cycle (C), in keeping with the 'machinery' murmur on auscultation

Slide 97 *Aortic coarctation* The membrane can be imaged from the suprasternal approach. Using pulsed Doppler, an increase in peak velocity can be shown as the sample volume approaches (A and B) then crosses (C) the defect. In a more severe defect, there is forward flow throughout diastole

Normal variants

Slide 98 *Subaortic bulging* This is a normal feature in patients aged over 60. There is localized subaortic bulging (arrows) but the rest of the left ventricle is of normal thickness. Hypertrophic cardiomyopathy should not be overdiagnosed

Slide 99 *Left ventricular tendon* Occasionally this is mistaken for an apical thrombus

Slide 100 *Prominent Eustachian valve* This valve (arrows) marks the opening of the inferior vena cava and is occasionally misdiagnosed as a right atrial mass

Slide 101 *Chiari network* This consists of a single strand or a fenestrated membrane (arrows) attached between the opening of the inferior vena cava, the atrial free wall and the atrial septum. It is caused by incomplete resorption of the embryological valve from which the valves at the opening of the inferior vena cava and the coronary sinus are derived. It is found in around 1% of all transthoracic studies

Cardiac source of emboli

Slide 102 *Left atrial ball thrombus* Rheumatic mitral stenosis associated with atrial fibrillation has an 18-fold relative risk of stroke. Usually overt thrombus is not imaged transthoracically and treatment with warfarin should be considered. However, on occasions, a ball thrombus is shown for which treatment is urgent surgery. Ball thrombus can cause stroke, syncope or sudden death

Slide 103 *Left atrial thrombus on transesophageal examination* Left atrial thrombi, for example this appendage thrombus (arrow), are found in approximately 10% of patients after a cerebral infarction compared with approximately 2% in normal control subjects. Other causes of stroke include endocarditis (Slide 32), aortic atheroma (Slide 92) and aortic dissection (Slide 89)

Slide 104 *Myxoma* Myxoma may present with stroke or with exertional breathlessness, syncope or with non-specific symptoms mimicking an occult malignancy or connective tissue disease. The clinical signs may suggest mitral valve disease. Echocardiographically, a myxoma is characterized by its attachment to the atrial septum and is frequently of mixed echogenicity. It lies within the left atrium during systole (a) but prolapses through the mitral valve in diastole (b)

Slide 105 *Patent foramen ovale on a transesophageal study* This is found in around 20% of patients with a cerebral infarction and in up to 50% in whom no other possible cause, such as carotid atheroma, can be found. In (a) there is an aneurysmal atrial septum. In (b) an injection of agitated air and blood in normal saline has been made into a large antecubital fossa vein. A flurry of contrast crosses into the left atrium during the first cycle (b) and more on successive cycles (c)

Key to figure abbreviations

Ao	aorta
Cx	circumflex
LA	left atrium
LAD	left anterior descending
LV	left ventricle
P	pericardium
PA	pulmonary artery
PW	posterior wall
RA	right atrium
RCA	right coronary artery
RV	right ventricle